# Contents

# Chapter 1: Introduction to Essential Oils

Essential oils have been gaining popularity for their aromatic and therapeutic properties, offering a natural and holistic approach to health and well-being. In this chapter, we'll delve into the basics, exploring what essential oils are, tracing their historical roots, and understanding the myriad benefits they offer to beginners entering the captivating world of aromatherapy.

## What are Essential Oils?

Essential oils are highly concentrated, volatile compounds extracted from various parts of plants, including leaves, flowers, bark, stems, and roots. These oils capture the plant's fragrance and other beneficial properties, giving them a distinctive scent and a range of potential health benefits. The extraction methods include steam distillation, cold pressing, or solvent extraction, ensuring the purity of the final product.

Each essential oil contains a unique combination of chemical constituents, making them versatile in addressing a wide array of physical, emotional, and mental concerns. From lavender's calming effects to peppermint's invigorating aroma, these oils have been used for centuries across different cultures for their therapeutic properties.

## History of Essential Oils

The history of essential oils can be traced back to ancient civilizations, where various cultures recognized the potent properties of aromatic plants. The Egyptians, Greeks, Romans, and Chinese were among the early practitioners of essential oil use for medicinal, religious, and cosmetic purposes.

The Egyptians, for example, employed essential oils in the embalming process, highlighting their belief in the oils' preservation and purification qualities. Meanwhile, the Greeks and Romans utilized essential oils in their bathhouses and massages for relaxation and rejuvenation.

During the Middle Ages, essential oils continued to play a crucial role in treating various ailments. The practice of distillation evolved, contributing to the refinement of extraction methods.

However, it was not until the 19th century that essential oils regained popularity in Western cultures with the development of modern aromatherapy.

Renowned figures like René-Maurice Gattefossé and Jean Valnet played pivotal roles in reintroducing the therapeutic benefits of essential oils. Gattefossé's work, particularly after his accidental discovery of lavender's healing properties, laid the foundation for the systematic use of essential oils in the field of aromatherapy.

**Benefits of Essential Oils**

Essential oils offer a surplus of benefits that extend beyond their pleasant aromas. Their therapeutic properties have made them valuable assets in promoting physical, emotional, and mental well-being. Here are some key benefits for beginners to explore:

1. Stress Relief and Relaxation:

   Essential oils like lavender, chamomile, and bergamot are renowned for their calming properties. Inhaling their aromas or incorporating them into massage oils can help alleviate stress and induce a sense of relaxation.


2. Improved Sleep:

Many essential oils, such as lavender, cedarwood, and frankincense, possess sleep-inducing qualities. Diffusing these oils in the bedroom or adding a few drops to a pillow can contribute to a restful night's sleep.


3. Boosted Mood and Energy:

Citrus oils like lemon, orange, and grapefruit are known for their uplifting scents. Inhaling these oils can enhance mood and increase energy levels, making them excellent choices for combating feelings of fatigue.


4. Skin Care and Healing:

Tea tree, lavender, and chamomile essential oils have skin-nourishing and healing properties. Diluting these oils in carrier oils or skincare products can contribute to healthier-looking skin and aid in addressing various skin concerns.

5. Respiratory Support:

Eucalyptus, peppermint, and tea tree oils are commonly used to support respiratory health. Inhaling their vapors or using them in steam inhalation can help ease congestion and promote clearer breathing.

6. Natural Cleaning Solutions:

Essential oils with antimicrobial properties, such as tea tree, lemon, and eucalyptus, can be incorporated into homemade cleaning solutions. Their natural disinfectant qualities make them effective alternatives to conventional cleaning products.

7. Pain Relief:

Some essential oils, like peppermint and eucalyptus, have analgesic properties that can help alleviate pain and discomfort. Mixing these oils with a carrier oil and applying the blend topically may provide relief for sore muscles or headaches.

8. Emotional Well-being:

Essential oils can have a profound impact on emotional health. Oils like ylang-ylang, rose, and frankincense are often used to promote a sense of emotional balance and well-being.

This introduction to essential oils provides a glimpse into the captivating world of aromatherapy, from their origins in ancient civilizations to the diverse benefits they offer. As you embark on your journey with essential oils, keep in mind that their effectiveness varies from person to person. Experimenting with different oils and methods of use will allow you to discover the unique benefits that resonate with you. In the upcoming chapters, we'll delve deeper into the specifics of using essential oils for various purposes, guiding you towards a more profound understanding of their applications in everyday life.

# Chapter 2: Understanding Essential Oils

In this chapter, we'll delve into the intricacies of essential oils, exploring the methods used for their extraction, the importance of quality and purity, and essential safety precautions that every enthusiast, especially beginners, should be aware of.

**Extraction Methods**

The extraction of essential oils is a meticulous process that involves obtaining the volatile compounds from plant material. Various extraction methods are employed, each suited to different types of plants and yielding oils with distinct characteristics. Here are some commonly used extraction methods:

1. Steam Distillation:

   Steam distillation is the most common method for extracting essential oils. It involves passing steam through the plant material, which causes the essential oil to evaporate. The steam and oil vapors are then condensed back into a liquid, with the oil floating on top of the water. This method is suitable for a wide range of plant materials and is known for producing high-quality essential oils.

## 2. Cold Pressing:

This method is primarily used for extracting essential oils from citrus fruits like lemons, oranges, and grapefruits. The rinds of the fruits are mechanically pressed to release the essential oil. Cold pressing is a simple and effective method, but it's limited to oils from fruits with easily extractable oils in their peels.

## 3. Solvent Extraction:

In solvent extraction, a solvent, often hexane, is used to dissolve the essential oil from the plant material. After extraction, the solvent is evaporated, leaving behind the essential oil. This method is suitable for delicate flowers that may be damaged by the heat of steam distillation. However, it's crucial to ensure that no solvent residue remains in the final product.

4. CO2 Extraction:

CO2 extraction utilizes carbon dioxide in a supercritical state to extract essential oils. This method allows for the extraction of a broader range of compounds and is often used for delicate and heat-sensitive plant materials. CO2 extraction tends to yield oils with a closer chemical composition to the original plant, making them highly sought after for therapeutic purposes.

Understanding the extraction method used for a particular essential oil can provide insights into its composition and potential benefits.

## Quality and Purity

The quality and purity of essential oils are paramount for ensuring their effectiveness and safety. With the growing popularity of aromatherapy, it's crucial for consumers, especially beginners, to be discerning when selecting essential oils. Here are key factors to consider:

1. Botanical Name and Source:

Always check the botanical name of the essential oil and its source. Different species of plants can yield oils with varying properties. Reputable manufacturers provide this information on the product label or packaging.

2. Purity Testing:

Look for oils that undergo third-party purity testing. This ensures that the oil is free from contaminants, additives, or diluents. The testing process typically includes gas chromatography and mass spectrometry to analyze the chemical composition of the oil.

3. Organic Certification:

Opt for organic essential oils when possible. Organic certification ensures that the plants were grown without synthetic pesticides or fertilizers, resulting in a purer final product. However, it's essential to note that not all high-quality oils are certified organic.

4. Sourcing and Distillation:

Consider the geographical origin of the plants and the distillation process. Some regions are known for producing oils with unique characteristics. Additionally, oils that undergo proper distillation, with the right temperature and duration, maintain their therapeutic properties.

5. Packaging:

The packaging of essential oils is crucial in preserving their quality. Oils should be stored in dark glass bottles to protect them from light, which can cause degradation. Airtight seals prevent exposure to air, helping to maintain the oil's freshness.

6. Price and Quality Relationship:

While cost may not always be an indicator of quality, extremely low-priced oils may be suspect. Quality essential oils require a significant amount of plant material to produce, and the price often reflects the labour-intensive extraction process.

Investing in high-quality, pure essential oils ensures that you receive the maximum therapeutic benefits without compromising on safety.

**Safety Precautions**

While essential oils offer numerous benefits, it's crucial to approach their use with caution, especially if you are a beginner. Adhering to safety precautions helps prevent adverse reactions and ensures a positive experience. Here are essential safety guidelines:

1. Dilution:

   Essential oils are highly concentrated and should be diluted before applying them to the skin. Carrier oils, such as jojoba, almond, or coconut oil, can be used to dilute essential oils. A common dilution ratio is 2-3 drops of essential oil per teaspoon of carrier oil.

2. Patch Testing:

   Before widespread use, perform a patch test by applying a diluted mixture of the essential oil to a small area of skin. Monitor for any adverse reactions, such as redness, itching, or irritation. If a reaction occurs, discontinue use.

### 3. Phototoxic Oils:

Some essential oils, particularly citrus oils like bergamot, lime, and lemon, can cause skin sensitivity to sunlight. Avoid exposure to direct sunlight or UV rays for 12-24 hours after applying these oils topically.

### 4. Pregnancy and Children:

Pregnant women and young children may be more sensitive to certain essential oils. Consult with a healthcare professional before using essential oils during pregnancy, and use caution when using oils around infants and young children.

### 5. Internal Use:

Not all essential oils are safe for internal use. Some can be toxic when ingested. Follow guidelines from reputable sources and consult with a qualified aromatherapist or healthcare professional before ingesting any essential oils.


## 6. Allergies and Sensitivities:

Individuals with allergies or sensitivities should exercise caution when using essential oils. Conduct patch tests and consult with a healthcare professional if there are concerns about potential allergic reactions.


## 7. Storage:

Store essential oils in a cool, dark place away from direct sunlight and heat. Proper storage helps maintain the oils' integrity and extends their shelf life.


## 8. Consultation with Healthcare Professionals:

If you have underlying health conditions or are taking medications, it's advisable to consult with a healthcare professional before incorporating essential oils into your wellness routine.

Understanding essential oils involves exploring their extraction methods, ensuring their quality and purity, and adhering to safety precautions. This knowledge forms the foundation for a positive and enriching experience with essential oils. As we move forward in this exploration, the subsequent chapters will delve into specific essential oils, their applications, and advanced techniques for harnessing their full potential. Remember, the journey with essential oils is a personal one, and by arming yourself with knowledge, you empower yourself to make informed and safe choices on this aromatic adventure.

# Chapter 3: Essential Oils and Their Properties

In this chapter, we'll explore the properties and diverse applications of some popular essential oils, each possessing unique characteristics that contribute to their therapeutic benefits. From the soothing aroma of lavender to the invigorating scent of peppermint, these essential oils play a significant role in aromatherapy and holistic well-being.

**Lavender Essential Oil**

Botanical Name: Lavandula angustifolia

Aroma: Floral, sweet, herbaceous

Properties:

- Calming and Relaxing: Lavender essential oil is renowned for its ability to promote relaxation and alleviate stress. Diffusing lavender oil in the bedroom or adding a few drops to a warm bath can contribute to a serene atmosphere.

- Sleep Aid: Known for its sedative properties, lavender oil is a popular choice for those seeking a natural sleep aid. A few drops on a pillow or in a diffuser before bedtime can help induce a restful night's sleep.

- Skin Care: Lavender oil has soothing and healing properties, making it beneficial for various skin conditions. It can be diluted in a carrier oil and applied topically to soothe minor burns, cuts, and skin irritations.

- Anti-anxiety: Inhaling the aroma of lavender oil may help reduce anxiety and promote a sense of calm. Consider using it during meditation or moments of relaxation.

**Peppermint Essential Oil**

Botanical Name: Mentha × piperita

Aroma: Minty, cool, invigorating

Properties:

- Energizing: Peppermint oil is known for its invigorating and energizing properties. Inhaling its scent can help combat fatigue and boost mental alertness.

- Digestive Aid: Peppermint oil is often used to alleviate digestive issues such as indigestion and bloating. It can be diluted and massaged onto the abdomen or added to a cup of tea.

- Headache Relief: Applying a diluted peppermint oil blend to the temples may provide relief from headaches and migraines. The cooling sensation can help soothe tension.

- Respiratory Support: Inhaling peppermint oil vapor can help clear the respiratory tract, making it beneficial for individuals dealing with congestion or sinus issues.

**Eucalyptus Essential Oil**

Botanical Name: Eucalyptus globulus

Aroma: Fresh, camphoraceous, slightly woody

Properties:

- Respiratory Health: Eucalyptus oil is well-known for its respiratory benefits. Inhaling its vapors can help clear the airways and ease congestion, making it a popular choice during cold and flu season.

- Antimicrobial: Eucalyptus oil has antimicrobial properties, making it a valuable addition to homemade cleaning products. Its germ-fighting abilities contribute to a healthier living environment.

- Mental Clarity: The refreshing aroma of eucalyptus oil is invigorating and may help enhance mental clarity and focus. Diffusing the oil in a workspace can create a stimulating atmosphere.

- Muscle and Joint Relief: Eucalyptus oil, when diluted in a carrier oil, can be applied topically to soothe sore muscles and joints. It provides a cooling sensation that aids in relaxation.

**Tea Tree Essential Oil**

Botanical Name: Melaleuca alternifolia

Aroma: Medicinal, earthy, slightly camphoraceous

Properties:

- Antiseptic: Tea tree oil is prized for its powerful antiseptic properties. It can be applied topically to minor cuts, wounds, and skin blemishes to prevent infection and promote healing.

- Acne Treatment: Due to its antibacterial and anti-inflammatory properties, tea tree oil is a popular choice for treating acne. It can be diluted and applied to affected areas with a cotton swab.

- Fungal Infections: Tea tree oil is effective against fungal infections such as athlete's foot and nail fungus. Diluted in a carrier oil, it can be applied topically to affected areas.

- Scalp Health: Incorporating tea tree oil into hair care routines can help maintain a healthy scalp. It is known for addressing dandruff and promoting overall scalp well-being.

**Lemon Essential Oil**

Botanical Name: Citrus limon

Aroma: Bright, citrusy, uplifting

Properties:

- Mood Enhancement: Lemon oil is celebrated for its uplifting and mood-enhancing properties. Diffusing the oil can create a refreshing and invigorating atmosphere.

- Antibacterial: Lemon oil possesses antibacterial properties, making it a natural disinfectant. It can be added to cleaning solutions to create a fresh and germ-free environment.

- Digestive Aid: Inhaling the scent of lemon oil or adding a drop to water before meals may help stimulate digestion and alleviate indigestion.

- Skin Brightening: Lemon oil is known for its skin-brightening properties. When diluted in a carrier oil, it can be applied topically to reduce the appearance of dark spots and promote a more even skin tone.

**Frankincense Essential Oil:**

Botanical Name: Boswellia carterii

Aroma: Woody, earthy, resinous

Properties:

- Spiritual and Meditative: Frankincense has a long history of use in spiritual and meditative practices. Its grounding and calming properties make it a popular choice for rituals and ceremonies.

- Anti-inflammatory: Frankincense oil may have anti-inflammatory effects, making it beneficial for conditions such as arthritis. Diluting and massaging onto affected areas can provide relief.

- Skincare: Frankincense is valued for its rejuvenating effects on the skin. When diluted in a carrier oil, it can be applied to reduce the appearance of fine lines and wrinkles.

**Rosemary Essential Oil:**

Botanical Name: Rosmarinus officinalis

Aroma: Herbaceous, woody, camphoraceous

Properties:

- Cognitive Function: Rosemary oil is believed to enhance cognitive function and concentration. Diffusing the oil or inhaling its aroma may support mental clarity.

- Hair Health: Rosemary oil is known for promoting hair health. Adding a few drops to shampoo or massaging it into the scalp with a carrier oil can stimulate hair growth and improve overall scalp condition.

- Pain Relief: Rosemary oil may have analgesic properties, making it beneficial for relieving muscle and joint pain. It can be diluted and applied topically to affected areas.

**Chamomile Essential Oil:**

Botanical Name: Matricaria chamomilla (German Chamomile), Chamaemelum nobile (Roman Chamomile)

Aroma: Sweet, fruity, herbaceous (German Chamomile), Sweet, apple-like (Roman Chamomile)

Properties:

- Calming: Chamomile oils are renowned for their calming and soothing effects. Diffusing chamomile oil or adding it to a warm bath can promote relaxation.

- Skin Irritations: Chamomile oil has anti-inflammatory properties, making it beneficial for soothing skin irritations. It can be diluted and applied topically to areas of redness or inflammation.

- Sleep Aid: Chamomile is often used to promote sleep and alleviate insomnia. A few drops on a pillow or in a diffuser before bedtime can contribute to a restful night's sleep.


These essential oils represent just a small selection of the vast array available, each with its unique properties and potential benefits. As you explore the world of essential oils, it's essential to remember that individual responses may vary, and experimentation will help you discover the oils that resonate best with your needs and preferences.

 Understanding the properties of essential oils opens up a world of possibilities for enhancing your well-being. From the calming effects of lavender to the invigorating aroma of peppermint, these oils offer a natural and holistic approach to health. As you incorporate essential oils into your daily routine, pay attention to your body's responses and explore different blends to find what works best for you. In the following chapters, we will delve into specific applications of essential oils, providing practical tips for using them in various aspects of your life. Enjoy the journey into the aromatic realm of essential oils and the positive impact they can have on your overall wellness.

# Chapter 4: Using Essential Oils

In this chapter, we'll explore the various methods of using essential oils to harness their therapeutic benefits. Understanding how to apply essential oils through diffusion, topical application, inhalation, and, when appropriate, internal use, empowers individuals to integrate these aromatic wonders into their daily lives.

## Diffusion

Diffusion is one of the most popular and accessible ways to enjoy the aromatic benefits of essential oils. There are several methods of diffusion, each offering a unique experience:

1. Ultrasonic Diffusers:

Ultrasonic diffusers use water to disperse a fine mist of essential oil into the air. These devices also serve as humidifiers, contributing to a balanced indoor environment. Ultrasonic diffusion is gentle and suitable for most essential oils.

2. Nebulizing Diffusers:

Nebulizing diffusers break down essential oils into tiny particles and release them into the air without the use of heat or water. This method maintains the oil's integrity, providing a more concentrated and potent aroma. Nebulizing diffusers are ideal for therapeutic purposes.

3. Evaporative Diffusers:

Evaporative diffusers use a fan or a porous material to release essential oil molecules into the air. While they are effective, the intensity of the aroma may vary, and some oils with volatile components may evaporate more quickly.

4. Heat Diffusers:

Heat diffusers utilize heat to evaporate essential oils into the air. While these are simple and cost-effective, the heat can alter the chemical composition of the oils, potentially diminishing their therapeutic properties.

**Tips for Diffusion:**

- Start with a few drops of essential oil and adjust based on your preference and the size of the space.

- Experiment with different oil combinations to create custom blends for various moods or purposes.

- Be mindful of the duration of diffusion to prevent olfactory fatigue—switch oils periodically.


**Topical Application**

Topical application involves applying diluted essential oils directly to the skin. Dilution is essential to prevent skin irritation, especially for those with sensitive skin. Here are some common methods of topical application:

1. Massage:

Combining essential oils with a carrier oil for massage allows for absorption through the skin. This method is not only relaxing but also facilitates the oils' penetration for systemic benefits.

2. Compress:

   Adding a few drops of essential oil to warm or cold water for a compress can be soothing for localized discomfort. A cloth is soaked in the water and applied to the affected area.

3. Bath:

   Adding a few drops of essential oil to a warm bath provides a luxurious and aromatic experience. Ensure proper dilution with a carrier oil or an emulsifier to disperse the oil evenly in the water.

4. Roller Bottles:

   Roller bottles are pre-diluted essential oil blends in a convenient roll-on applicator. These are easy to carry and can be applied to pulse points for quick and targeted use.

**Tips for Topical Application:**

- Always perform a patch test before widespread use to check for skin sensitivity.

- Follow recommended dilution ratios, typically ranging from 1% to 3% for adults, depending on the purpose and essential oil.

- Pay attention to application areas, avoiding sensitive areas such as the eyes and mucous membranes.

**Inhalation**

Inhalation involves directly inhaling the aroma of essential oils, allowing their molecules to interact with the olfactory system and, in turn, the brain. There are various methods of inhalation:

1. Direct Inhalation:

Inhaling the scent directly from the bottle or by placing a few drops on a tissue allows for quick and immediate access to the aromatic benefits. This method is convenient and can be used throughout the day.

2. Steam Inhalation:

Adding a few drops of essential oil to a bowl of hot water and inhaling the steam is effective for respiratory support. This method can help alleviate congestion and promote clearer breathing.

3. Aromatherapy Jewelry:

Diffuser jewelry, such as necklaces or bracelets with absorbent pads, allows individuals to carry the aroma of their favorite essential oils throughout the day.

4. Personal Inhalers:

Portable inhalers contain a wick that can be infused with essential oils. These are discreet and convenient for on-the-go aromatherapy.

Tips for Inhalation:

- Practice deep, mindful breathing while inhaling essential oils for a more profound impact on the nervous system.

- Experiment with single oils or blends to find scents that resonate with your mood or goals.

- Consider using inhalation as a quick pick-me-up during moments of stress or fatigue.

**Internal Use**

Internal use of essential oils involves ingesting them in small amounts. It's essential to note that not all essential oils are safe for internal use, and this method should be approached with caution. Only therapeutic-grade oils labeled for internal use should be ingested, and guidance from a healthcare professional or certified aromatherapist is advisable.

1. Culinary Use:

Some essential oils, such as peppermint, lemon, and oregano, can be used in cooking to add flavour to dishes. A tiny amount goes a long way, and it's crucial to use oils specifically labelled as safe for consumption.

2. Capsules:

Creating homemade vegetable capsules with a carrier oil and a drop or two of essential oil is another method of internal use. This allows for precise control over the dosage.

**Tips for Internal Use:**

- Research and ensure that the specific essential oil is safe for internal consumption.

- Use high-quality, therapeutic-grade essential oils labelled for internal use.

- Start with minimal amounts and gradually increase if necessary.

- Seek guidance from a healthcare professional or qualified aromatherapist.

## Safety Precautions for All Methods

Regardless of the method of use, it's crucial to observe safety precautions to ensure a positive and safe experience with essential oils:

1. Dilution:

   Always dilute essential oils before applying them to the skin. This helps prevent skin irritation and sensitivity.

2. Quality Matters:

   Invest in high-quality, pure essential oils. Third-party testing and certification ensure that the oils are free from contaminants.

3. Pregnancy and Children:

   Pregnant women and young children may be more sensitive to certain essential oils. Consult with a healthcare professional before using oils during pregnancy or on children.

4. Allergies and Sensitivities:

Individuals with allergies or sensitivities should exercise caution when using essential oils. Perform patch tests and discontinue use if irritation occurs.

5. Storage:

Properly store essential oils in dark glass bottles in a cool, dry place away from direct sunlight and heat to maintain their integrity.

6. Educate Yourself:

Continuously educate yourself on the properties and safe use of essential oils. Stay informed about any contraindications or new research.

Understanding the various methods of using essential oils opens up a world of possibilities for integrating these potent plant extracts into your daily routine. Whether diffusing for a calming atmosphere, applying topically for targeted benefits, inhaling for a quick mood lift, or, when appropriate, using internally for specific health goals, essential oils offer a holistic approach to well-being. As you explore and experiment with different oils and methods, pay attention to your body's responses and enjoy the sensory journey that essential oils provide. The next chapters will delve into specific applications of essential oils in various aspects of life, providing practical tips and guidance for enhancing your overall wellness.

# Chapter 5: Essential Oil Recipes

In this chapter, we'll explore a collection of essential oil recipes designed to cater to various aspects of well-being, including relaxation, energy boost, sleep aid, and skincare. These blends and formulations allow you to harness the therapeutic benefits of essential oils in a practical and enjoyable way.

## 1. Relaxation Blend

Ingredients:

- 4 drops Lavender (Lavandula angustifolia)

- 3 drops Chamomile (Matricaria chamomilla)

- 2 drops Bergamot (Citrus bergamia)

- 1 drop Frankincense (Boswellia carterii)

- 2 tablespoons Carrier Oil (such as sweet almond or jojoba)

Instructions:

1. Mix the essential oils in a small, dark glass bottle.

2. Add the carrier oil to the blend and shake well to combine.

3. Use the relaxation blend for a calming massage or add a few drops to a diffuser before bedtime.

Benefits:

This blend promotes a sense of tranquility and relaxation, making it ideal for winding down after a long day or creating a peaceful atmosphere during meditation.


**2. Energy Boost Blend**

Ingredients:

- 4 drops Peppermint (Mentha × piperita)

- 3 drops Lemon (Citrus limon)

- 2 drops Rosemary (Rosmarinus officinalis)

- 1 drop Eucalyptus (Eucalyptus globulus)

- 2 tablespoons Carrier Oil


Instructions:

1. Combine the essential oils in a small, dark glass bottle.

2. Add the carrier oil and mix well.

3. Apply a small amount to pulse points or inhale the aroma directly from the bottle for a quick energy boost.

Benefits:

This invigorating blend provides a natural pick-me-up, promoting mental alertness and energy. Perfect for those midday slumps or whenever you need a revitalizing lift.


### 3. Sleep Aid Pillow Spray

Ingredients:

- 15 drops Lavender (Lavandula angustifolia)

- 10 drops Roman Chamomile (Chamaemelum nobile)

- 5 drops Cedarwood (Cedrus atlantica)

- 1.5 ounces Distilled Water


Instructions:

1. In a small spray bottle, combine the essential oils.

2. Add distilled water to the bottle and shake well before each use.

3. Lightly spritz your pillow and bedding before bedtime.

Benefits:

This calming pillow spray creates a serene sleep environment, helping to ease the mind and promote a restful night's sleep.

4. Nourishing Skin Serum

Ingredients:

- 5 drops Frankincense (Boswellia carterii)

- 5 drops Lavender (Lavandula angustifolia)

- 5 drops Geranium (Pelargonium graveolens)

- 1 ounce Jojoba Oil

Instructions:

1. Combine the essential oils in a dark glass dropper bottle.

2. Add jojoba oil to the blend and shake well.

3. Apply a few drops to clean, damp skin, focusing on areas that need extra nourishment.

Benefits:

This luxurious skin serum supports healthy skin, providing hydration and promoting a radiant complexion. Use it in your daily skincare routine for a natural glow.

## 5. Refreshing Citrus Body Scrub

Ingredients:

- 1 cup Epsom Salt

- 1/2 cup Fractionated Coconut Oil

- 10 drops Grapefruit (Citrus paradisi)

- 8 drops Orange (Citrus sinensis)

- 6 drops Lemon (Citrus limon)

Instructions:

1. In a mixing bowl, combine Epsom salt and fractionated coconut oil.

2. Add the essential oils and mix thoroughly.

3. Use the scrub in the shower, gently massaging onto damp skin in circular motions, and rinse.

Benefits:

This invigorating body scrub exfoliates and rejuvenates the skin, leaving you feeling refreshed and energized. The citrus essential oils provide a delightful aroma.

### 6. Soothing Aftershave Balm

Ingredients:

- 5 drops Tea Tree (Melaleuca alternifolia)

- 5 drops Lavender (Lavandula angustifolia)

- 2 drops Peppermint (Mentha × piperita)

- 2 tablespoons Aloe Vera Gel

Instructions:

1. In a small bowl, combine the essential oils.

2. Add the aloe vera gel and mix well.

3. Apply the soothing balm to freshly shaved skin.

Benefits:

This aftershave balm provides a cooling and soothing effect on the skin, reducing irritation and promoting a smooth post-shave experience.

## 7. Relaxing Bath Salt Blend

Ingredients:

- 1 cup Epsom Salt

- 1/2 cup Himalayan Pink Salt

- 10 drops Lavender (Lavandula angustifolia)

- 5 drops Ylang-Ylang (Cananga odorata)

- 5 drops Patchouli (Pogostemon cablin)

Instructions:

1. In a mixing bowl, combine Epsom salt and Himalayan pink salt.

2. Add the essential oils and mix thoroughly.

3. Add the bath salt blend to warm bathwater and enjoy a relaxing soak.

Benefits:

This indulgent bath salt blend enhances relaxation, soothes muscles, and provides an aromatic escape after a stressful day.

## 8. Mood-Boosting Room Spray

Ingredients:

- 15 drops Bergamot (Citrus bergamia)

- 10 drops Lemon (Citrus limon)

- 5 drops Clary Sage (Salvia sclarea)

- 2 ounces Distilled Water

Instructions:

1. In a small spray bottle, combine the essential oils.

2. Add distilled water to the bottle and shake well before each use.

3. Spritz the room spray in your living space to create a uplifting and mood-boosting atmosphere.

Benefits:

This room spray combines citrus and herbal notes to elevate the mood and create a positive ambiance in your home or workspace.

## Safety Precautions for Essential Oil Recipes

- Patch Test: Before widespread use, perform a patch test to check for any adverse reactions or skin sensitivities.

 - Dilution: Always dilute essential oils, especially for topical application, to prevent skin irritation.

- Quality Matters: Use high-quality, pure essential oils from reputable sources to ensure efficacy and safety.

- Pregnancy and Children: Consult with a healthcare professional before using essential oils during pregnancy or on young children.

- Storage: Keep essential oil blends in dark glass bottles in a cool, dry place away from direct sunlight.

- Educate Yourself: Stay informed about any contraindications or precautions related to specific essential oils.

These essential oil recipes offer a glimpse into the versatile and enjoyable world of aromatherapy. Whether you're seeking relaxation, an energy boost, improved sleep, or enhanced skincare, incorporating these blends into your daily routine can bring a sense of well-being and joy. As you explore and create your own formulations, remember to listen to your body's responses and tailor the recipes to suit your preferences.

# Chapter 6: Frequently Asked Questions

In this chapter, we'll address some common questions and concerns regarding the use of essential oils. From considerations during pregnancy to using oils on children and pets, these frequently asked questions aim to provide clarity and guidance for a safe and enjoyable experience with essential oils.

1. Can I use essential oils if I'm pregnant?

The use of essential oils during pregnancy requires caution and careful consideration. While some essential oils can be beneficial during this time, it's essential to be aware of potential risks and contraindications. Certain oils, especially those with strong chemical components, may be best avoided during pregnancy.

Guidelines:

- Consultation: Always consult with your healthcare provider before using essential oils during pregnancy. They can provide personalized advice based on your health history and specific circumstances.

- Avoid Certain Oils: Some essential oils, such as clary sage, rosemary, and basil, are generally advised to be avoided during the first trimester. Others, like lavender and chamomile, may be used with caution.

- Dilution: If using essential oils topically, ensure proper dilution to minimize the risk of skin irritation. A 1% dilution (1 drop of essential oil per teaspoon of carrier oil) is often recommended.

- Gentle Aromatherapy: Opt for gentle aromatherapy methods, such as diffusing, rather than direct topical application, especially during the first trimester.

## 2. Can essential oils be used on children?

Using essential oils on children requires careful consideration due to their developing and sensitive systems. While certain oils can be beneficial, others may pose risks. Here are some guidelines to follow:

Guidelines:

- Age Consideration: Essential oil use is generally not recommended for infants under three months. For older children, consider their age, weight, and overall health.

- Dilution: Always dilute essential oils when applying them topically on children. A 0.25% to 1% dilution is typically recommended.

- Kid-Friendly Oils: Opt for mild essential oils such as lavender, chamomile, and tea tree. Avoid potentially irritating or stimulating oils like peppermint and eucalyptus.

- Consultation: If in doubt, consult with a pediatrician or a qualified aromatherapist for guidance on specific oils and their appropriate dilution.


3. Can I use essential oils on my pets?

Using essential oils on pets requires caution, as animals can react differently than humans. Some essential oils may be toxic to certain animals, especially cats, and small dogs. Here are considerations for using essential oils on pets:

Guidelines:

- Research: Before using any essential oils around pets, research the specific oil to ensure it is safe for the type of pet you have. Cats, for example, are more sensitive to certain oils.

- Dilution: If using essential oils on pets, always dilute them significantly. A diffuser with proper ventilation is often safer than applying oils directly to a pet's fur or skin.

- Observe Reactions: Monitor your pet's reactions to essential oils. If you notice any signs of distress, discomfort, or unusual behavior, discontinue use and consult with a veterinarian.

- Avoid Certain Oils: Some oils, like tea tree and citrus oils, can be toxic to pets. Avoid using oils with high phenol content around animals.


## 4. Are essential oils safe for internal use?

The internal use of essential oils is a topic of debate within the aromatherapy community. While some oils are considered safe for culinary purposes, not all essential oils are suitable for internal use. Here are some considerations:

Guidelines:

- Quality Matters: If considering internal use, ensure you are using high-quality, therapeutic-grade essential oils that are labeled for internal consumption.

- Dosage: Internal use should be approached with caution, and minimal amounts should be used. A drop or two diluted in a carrier oil or added to food is often sufficient.

- Consultation: Consult with a healthcare professional or a qualified aromatherapist before using essential oils internally, especially if you have underlying health conditions.

- Avoid Certain Oils: Some oils are not suitable for internal use due to their chemical composition. Oils high in phenols or aldehydes, for example, may be irritating to the digestive system.

## 5. Can essential oils interact with medications?

It's crucial to be aware that essential oils can potentially interact with medications. While many people use essential oils safely alongside their medications, there are considerations to keep in mind:

Guidelines:

- Consultation: Inform your healthcare provider about your use of essential oils, especially if you are taking medications. They can advise on potential interactions or contraindications.

- Citrus Oils: Some citrus essential oils, such as grapefruit and bergamot, may interact with certain medications by affecting enzyme activity in the liver. Exercise caution with these oils.

- Anticoagulant Medications: People taking anticoagulant medications should be cautious with essential oils high in coumarins, such as cinnamon and sweet orange.

- Blood Pressure Medications: Certain essential oils, like clary sage and ylang-ylang, may influence blood pressure. Consult with a healthcare professional if you have concerns.

6. Can essential oils cause skin irritation?

Skin irritation is a common concern when using essential oils, especially if applied undiluted. Some oils are more likely to cause irritation than others. Here are some guidelines to prevent skin irritation:

Guidelines:

- Dilution: Always dilute essential oils before applying them to the skin. Carrier oils, such as jojoba or sweet almond oil, can be used for dilution.

- Patch Test: Before widespread use, perform a patch test by applying a small amount of the diluted oil to a small area of skin. Monitor for any signs of irritation over 24 hours.

- Sensitive Skin: Individuals with sensitive skin should be especially cautious and consider using oils known for their gentle properties, such as lavender and chamomile.

- Photosensitive Oils: Some oils, particularly citrus oils, can cause skin sensitivity to sunlight. Avoid sun exposure after applying these oils to the skin.

7. Are all essential oils safe for diffusing?

While diffusing essential oils is a popular and safe method of use, not all oils are suitable for this application. Some oils may have strong aromas that could be overpowering, while others may have potential respiratory effects. Consider the following:

Guidelines:

- Moderation: Use essential oils in moderation when diffusing. A few drops are often sufficient to fill a room with the desired aroma.

- Respiratory Sensitivity: Individuals with respiratory sensitivities may need to be cautious with certain oils, particularly those high in camphor or cineole, such as eucalyptus.

- Citrus Oils: Citrus oils are generally safe for diffusion, but individuals with photosensitivity concerns may want to be mindful of exposure to sunlight.

- Quality Diffuser: Invest in a quality diffuser that is easy to clean and properly disperses the essential oil into the air.

8. Can essential oils help with headaches?

Essential oils are often used to alleviate headaches and migraines. Certain oils

have properties that may help ease tension and promote relaxation. Here are some considerations:

Guidelines:

- Peppermint: Peppermint oil is commonly used for headache relief. Dilute a drop of peppermint oil in a carrier oil and apply to the temples and back of the neck.

- Lavender: Lavender oil is known for its calming properties. Diffusing lavender or applying diluted lavender oil to the temples may provide relief.

- Frankincense: Frankincense oil may help alleviate stress-related headaches. Diffuse frankincense or inhale the aroma for a calming effect.

- Personal Preferences: Individual responses vary, so it may take some experimentation to find the oils that work best for your headache relief.

9. Can essential oils be used for respiratory support?

Essential oils can be beneficial for respiratory support, especially during times of congestion or seasonal discomfort. Here are some considerations:

Guidelines:

- Eucalyptus: Eucalyptus oil is well-known for its respiratory benefits. Use in a steam inhalation or diffuse to promote clear breathing.

- Tea Tree: Tea tree oil has antimicrobial properties and may be helpful for respiratory support. Diffuse or add a drop to a bowl of hot water for steam inhalation.

- Peppermint: Peppermint oil has a refreshing aroma and may help open up the airways. Diffuse or inhale for respiratory relief.

- Cautions: Be cautious with strong oils and consider individual sensitivities. Always follow proper dilution guidelines for topical application.

10. How do I choose high-quality essential oils?

Choosing high-quality essential oils is essential for a safe and effective aromatherapy experience. With numerous brands and options available, consider the following criteria when selecting essential oils:

Guidelines:

- Purity: Look for oils that are labelled as 100% pure and free from additives or synthetic ingredients. Check for third-party testing or certifications.

- Botanical Name: Reputable brands provide the botanical name of each oil, ensuring clarity about the plant species.

- Extraction Method: The extraction method can impact the quality of the oil. Cold-pressing and steam distillation are common methods that preserve the integrity of the oil.

- Packaging: Essential oils should be stored in dark glass bottles to protect them from light degradation. Avoid oils in clear or plastic containers.

- Reputation: Choose oils from reputable brands with a history of transparency, quality, and positive customer reviews.


Navigating the world of essential oils involves understanding their properties, applications, and potential interactions. By addressing common questions and concerns, this chapter aims to provide clarity and guidance for a safe and enjoyable experience with essential oils. Always prioritize safety, be aware of individual sensitivities, and consult with healthcare professionals when needed. As you incorporate essential oils into your daily life, remember that the journey is personal, and finding what works best for you involves exploration and experimentation. The next chapter will delve into advanced techniques and applications for those looking to deepen their understanding of essential oils.

# Chapter 7: Conclusion

As we conclude our journey through the world of essential oils, it's evident that these aromatic extracts have woven themselves into the fabric of holistic well-being. From their historical roots to their diverse applications in modern lifestyles, essential oils offer a sensory journey that encompasses physical, emotional, and mental realms. This chapter serves as a reflection on the path we've explored and a glimpse into the evolving landscape of essential oils.

**The Future of Essential Oils**

The future of essential oils is promising, marked by ongoing research, innovation, and an increasing awareness of their potential benefits. As scientific understanding deepens, we can anticipate more precise knowledge about the therapeutic properties of individual oils and their specific applications. Integrating essential oils into mainstream healthcare and wellness practices is a trend that continues to gain momentum.

1. Scientific Advancements:

Ongoing research is uncovering the intricate mechanisms through which essential oils interact with the body. This includes exploring their effects on neurotransmitters, immune responses, and cellular processes. As scientific methodologies advance, we can expect a more comprehensive understanding of how essential oils contribute to overall well-being.

2. Personalized Aromatherapy:

The future may bring about a more personalized approach to aromatherapy, tailoring essential oil recommendations based on an individual's unique preferences, health conditions, and genetic factors. This personalized approach could optimize the therapeutic benefits of essential oils for each person.

3. Integration into Healthcare:

Essential oils are increasingly finding their place in healthcare settings. From aromatherapy in hospitals to the inclusion of essential oils in complementary therapies, healthcare professionals are recognizing the potential of these natural extracts to enhance patient well-being.

4. Sustainable Sourcing:

   With growing awareness of environmental conservation and sustainability, the future of essential oils involves a focus on responsible sourcing. Ethical practices, fair trade initiatives, and sustainable cultivation methods will likely play a significant role in shaping the industry.

5. Innovative Applications:

   As essential oils continue to capture the interest of diverse industries, we may witness innovative applications beyond traditional use. This could include the integration of essential oils in beauty products, culinary experiences, and even in advanced medical treatments.

**Further Reading and Resources**

For those inspired to deepen their understanding of essential oils and explore their versatile applications, a wealth of resources is available. Whether you are a novice or a seasoned enthusiast, the following recommendations provide a roadmap for continued exploration:

1. Books:

   - "The Complete Book of Essential Oils and Aromatherapy" by Valerie Ann Worwood: A comprehensive guide covering essential oils, their properties, and practical applications for health and well-being.

   - "Aromatherapy for Healing the Spirit" by Gabriel Mojay: Explores the emotional and spiritual aspects of aromatherapy, offering insights into the profound effects of essential oils on the psyche.

   - "Essential Oil Safety" by Robert Tisserand and Rodney Young: An in-depth resource on the safety considerations of using essential oils, including proper dilution and contraindications.

2. Websites and Online Platforms:

   - National Association for Holistic Aromatherapy (NAHA): (https://naha.org/) NAHA provides valuable information on aromatherapy, including educational resources, safety guidelines, and a directory of certified aromatherapists.

   - Aromatherapy United: (https://aromatherapyunited.org/) An online community that fosters discussions, shares resources, and provides a platform for connecting with other aromatherapy enthusiasts.

   - PubMed: (https://pubmed.ncbi.nlm.nih.gov/) For those interested in scientific research, PubMed is a database of peer-reviewed articles on essential oils and aromatherapy.

 3. Courses and Workshops:

   - Institute of Traditional Herbal Medicine and Aromatherapy (ITHMA): (https://aromatherapy-studies.com/) Offers professional courses and workshops in aromatherapy and herbal medicine.

   - Aromahead Institute: (https://www.aromahead.com/) Provides online courses, webinars, and resources for individuals looking to deepen their knowledge of aromatherapy.

4. Certifications and Associations:

- Alliance of International Aromatherapists (AIA): (https://www.alliance-aromatherapists.org/) AIA is a professional organization that promotes education and ethical practices in aromatherapy. They offer resources and certification programs.

- International Federation of Professional Aromatherapists (IFPA): (https://www.ifparoma.org/) IFPA is a global organization that sets standards for aromatherapy education and practice. They offer certifications and resources for practitioners.

**Final Thoughts**

The world of essential oils is as diverse and dynamic as the aromatic compounds they contain. From the soothing notes of lavender to the invigorating scents of citrus, essential oils have the power to elevate our sensory experiences and contribute to a holistic approach to well-being.

As you embark on your journey with essential oils, remember that the key to a fulfilling and safe experience lies in knowledge, respect, and a mindful exploration of the vast botanical landscape. Whether you are seeking relaxation, energy, skincare, or emotional balance, essential oils offer a natural and aromatic path to enhance your daily life.

May your aromatic journey continue to unfold, filled with the delightful scents of nature and the therapeutic embrace of essential oils. As you explore the possibilities and weave these aromatic threads into the tapestry of your life, may you find moments of serenity, vitality, and joy.

Wishing you a fragrant and fulfilling journey with essential oils!